DEDICATION

This book is dedicated to my mom, Jenny. You are the strongest woman I know. Thank you for your strength. I will love you always.

TABLE OF CONTENTS

Conceive a Baby Naturally

The Least Expensive but Most Effective Way of Getting Pregnant

By: Monica Libinski

9781681272580

PUBLISHERS NOTES

Disclaimer – Speedy Publishing LLC

This publication is intended to provide helpful and informative material. It is not intended to diagnose, treat, cure, or prevent any health problem or condition, nor is intended to replace the advice of a physician. No action should be taken solely on the contents of this book. Always consult your physician or qualified health-care professional on any matters regarding your health and before adopting any suggestions in this book or drawing inferences from it.

The author and publisher specifically disclaim all responsibility for any liability, loss or risk, personal or otherwise, which is incurred as a consequence, directly or indirectly, from the use or application of any contents of this book.

Any and all product names referenced within this book are the trademarks of their respective owners. None of these owners have sponsored, authorized, endorsed, or approved this book.

Always read all information provided by the manufacturers' product labels before using their products. The author and publisher are not responsible for claims made by manufacturers.

This book was originally printed before 2014. This is an adapted reprint by Speedy Publishing LLC with newly updated content designed to help readers with much more accurate and timely information and data.

Speedy Publishing LLC

40 E Main Street, Newark, Delaware, 19711

Contact Us: 1-888-248-4521

Website: http://www.speedypublishing.co

REPRINTED Paperback Edition: 9781681272580:

Manufactured in the United States of America

Chapter 1- Why Can't You Bear a Child?

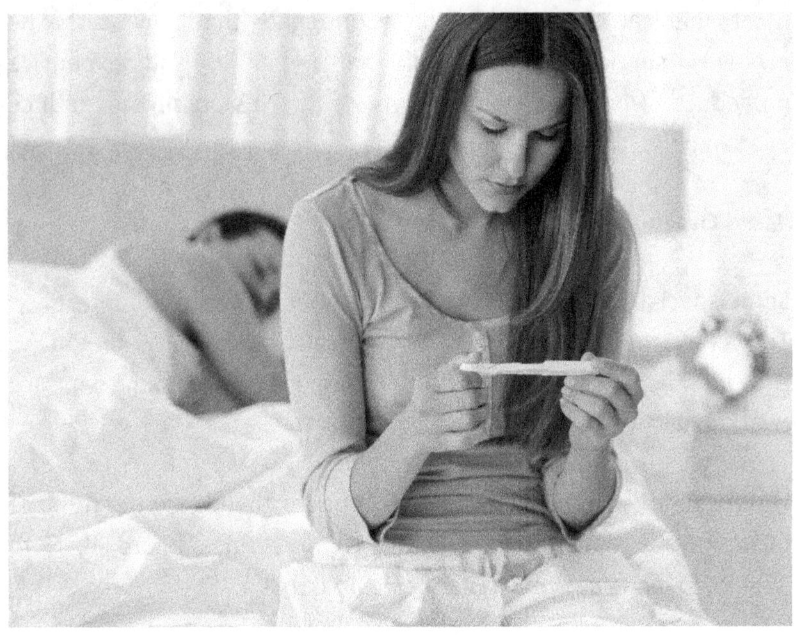

Why Can't a Woman Become a Mother?

There are so many different reasons for infertility, in both men and women, that it's impossible to use a blanket term to cover everything. Instead, it's important to look at various things that could affect your chances of conceiving and consider what diagnosis suits your own personal situation.

Ovarian Cysts

Ovarian cysts are small fluid-filled sacs that develop in the ovaries. In most cases, they're completely harmless, but they can rupture and cause tremendous pain. If a ruptured cyst is left untreated, it can form sepsis, which is quite toxic and potentially lethal.

Of course, the presence of ovarian cysts can also interfere with normal conception.

Most medical specialists will recommend that any cysts be removed surgically, which can be a painful and expensive procedure. What they don't tell you is that it's possible to reduce ovarian cysts naturally and painlessly.

'Lazy' Ovaries

Some specialists will diagnose 'lazy' ovaries as a cause of infertility. This simply means an egg isn't being released when it should, so they'll tend to prescribe infertility drugs, such as Clomid, to induce ovulation.

Unfortunately, studies in Washington have proved that the number of women who had taken Clomid is three times more likely to develop ovarian cancer than those who don't.

Once again, these specialists forget to let you know there are ways to stimulate and induce ovulation using natural methods. Of course, when you consider that the infertility drug industry is now a billion dollar industry, why would they want you to know you could do it yourself?

PCOS (Polycystic Ovarian Syndrome)

Polycystic Ovarian Syndrome is the term given when many small cysts are apparent within the ovaries. PCOS is thought to be one of the leading causes of female infertility. In some cases, this can be linked to obesity, acne, increased insulin resistance, lack of ovulation and sometimes an excess of masculinizing hormones.

Of course, this doesn't mean every patient who has acne or who is obese will have PCOS. Similarly, patients who have ovarian cysts may not have PCOS.

Similarly, patients showing an excess of masculinizing hormones may show unwanted facial and body hair growth as well as developing acne, but they also may not have PCOS.

Correct diagnosis can sometimes be difficult, but treatment can be relatively easy with prescription of a dietary supplement known as DCI, which is a naturally occurring human metabolite that helps with insulin metabolism.

Endometriosis

Endometriosis is the medical name given when the uterine lining that would normally shed as part of a regular monthly menstrual cycle grows on the outside of the uterus instead of inside. This is a major cause of infertility in women.

Endometriosis can cause very painful menstrual periods, as well as heavy bleeding and can be responsible for repeated miscarriages.

Infertility Specialists recommend laparoscopic surgery to remove the endometrial lining and any abnormal tissue; however, there are plenty of alternative natural therapies available to remedy this problem.

There are plenty of success stories from patients with endometriosis using traditional Chinese medicine, including traditional herbalism and acupuncture.

Fallopian Tube Blockages

Blocked or damaged fallopian tubes are thought to account for up to 40% of female infertility problems. Blocked tubes will prevent eggs reaching the uterus and prevent sperm from reaching the egg. In most cases, women have no idea their tubes might be blocked, as there are generally no obvious symptoms to look for. Blocked fallopian tubes are generally diagnosed by pelvic ultrasound, although a hysterosalpinogram may also be used, in which a dye is placed into the cervix before x-raying the pelvic region.

There are two types of blocked tubes – partial blockage and Hydro salpinx.

A partial blockage may be a result of endometrial lining closing off a portion of the tube, which can result in a tubal pregnancy, or ectopic pregnancy. A hydro salpinx is when the tube is completely blocked and begins to fill with fluid, which makes the tube dilate and swell as it fills. If both tubes are affected, the chances of conceiving are zero.

The predominant causes of blocked tubes are a history of Pelvic Inflammatory Disease, Chlamydia, ruptured appendix, endometriosis or other type of uterine infection.

Infertility specialists will advise that laparoscopic surgery is required to unblock the affected tubes; however this can cause further scarring in some cases. In the case of a hydro salpinx, a specialist may advise that a hydro salpingectomy is required, which is complete removal of the dilated fallopian tube. This destroys any chance of falling pregnant naturally in future and the patient becomes dependent on IVF treatments if further children are wanted.

Once again, there are plenty of non-surgical options available to help unblock damaged fallopian tubes. Alternative therapies that include manual physical therapy have also shown positive results.

Why a Man Can't Father a Child?

Most people are simply unaware that around 35-40% of all infertility problems are because of the male. It's almost instantly assumed that the female must be having some kind of problems.

Yet male infertility is almost as high as female infertility. Some of the common causes of male infertility are widely recognized, such as low sperm count, but there are others that aren't quite so well-known.

Low Sperm Count

Low sperm count or poor sperm mobility can cause infertility. There are many biological and environmental factors that can cause a low sperm count.

Age is a factor in sperm production, with a 60% fertilization rate evident in men younger than 39, but only a 30% fertilization rate for men older than 40.

However, factors such as stress, impotence and premature ejaculation can reduce sperm counts as well. In these cases, it could be wise to work on ways to reduce stress levels and work on the mental and emotion causes behind impotence and premature ejaculation before considering medical treatments.

Substance abuse and smoking are well known to both impair sperm count and reduce mobility drastically. It's also been proven that men who smoke have far lower sex drives, so have sex less frequently.

Men who have poor diets or who have specific deficiencies in vitamin C, selenium, zinc or folate are at far greater risk for low sperm count.

Overheating the testicles can cause temporary low sperm counts and this can be caused by things like saunas, hot tubs, high fever or even wearing underwear that causes the testicles to sit too close to the heat of the body. Combat this by wearing boxer shorts.

Surprisingly, one of the leading causes of impotence and infertility in men is bicycling. This is because pressure from the bike seat can damage sensitive blood vessels and nerves that cause erections and conduct blood flow to the perineum (the area between the scrotum and the anus). This can damage the testicles and scrotum, reducing sperm production.

Infertility specialists will happily prescribe drugs and medication to increase sperm count and boost sperm production. Incidentally, these are similar to those that stimulate ovulation. Side effects of drugs such as clomiphene and hMG can cause blurred vision, weight gain and even liver damage.

Yet there are many, many natural ways to increase sperm count without resorting to drugs or medications.

Male Tube Blockages

Infertility in men can sometimes be caused by tubal blockages in the vas deferens or epididymis (these are the tubes that transport sperm).

The most common cause of male tube blockage is varicose veins within the testicles. However, some sexually transmitted diseases, such as Chlamydia or gonorrhea can also cause blockage problems.

Doctors will recommend surgery to repair the varicoceles, but it should be noted that it can take between 6 and 9 months before a male will be able to impregnate a woman after the surgery.

Once again, there are plenty of natural treatments that can help to rectify these problems, yet far too many people don't even consider them.

The "Non-Specified" Reason for Couple Infertility

Of course, there are a percentage of couples who are diagnosed with 'non-specific infertility'. These are the couples where nothing specific can be located to explain why conception isn't happening.

Despite months of trying to conceive and subsequent months of tests, trials and specialist's appointments, many couples still don't have a logical explanation for why they can't fall pregnant.

When OB-GYNs and infertility specialists run a battery of tests, they're medically based. They look for hormonal imbalances. They look for the obvious signs of blocked tubes, cysts, sperm quality and quantity and other usual signs that something might be wrong that they can fix with medications or surgery.

Unfortunately, when they can't find anything logical, it's categorized as 'non-specific infertility' and they tend to resort to putting the couple onto fertility drugs like Clomid to see if that will help.

What they forget is the enormous range of other factors that can affect fertility that have nothing to do with the obvious symptoms the majority of people tend to display.

Our bodies are designed to send out warning signals when something is wrong. These signals are usually displayed as pain or symptoms or other issues that need to be addressed in order to fix the cause.

Unfortunately, the multi-billion dollar pharmaceutical industry would much rather treat the symptoms rather than work on ways to fix the cause of the problem in the first place.

By taking pain relief medication, you're actually masking the real warning sign your body is trying to give you. By taking infertility drugs, you're denying that your body is sending out a message that something is wrong with your reproductive system that needs to be addressed first, before you conceive your child.

This can sometimes lead to making the original problem even worse in the long run.

Chapter 2- See Your Body as a Well-Oiled Machine

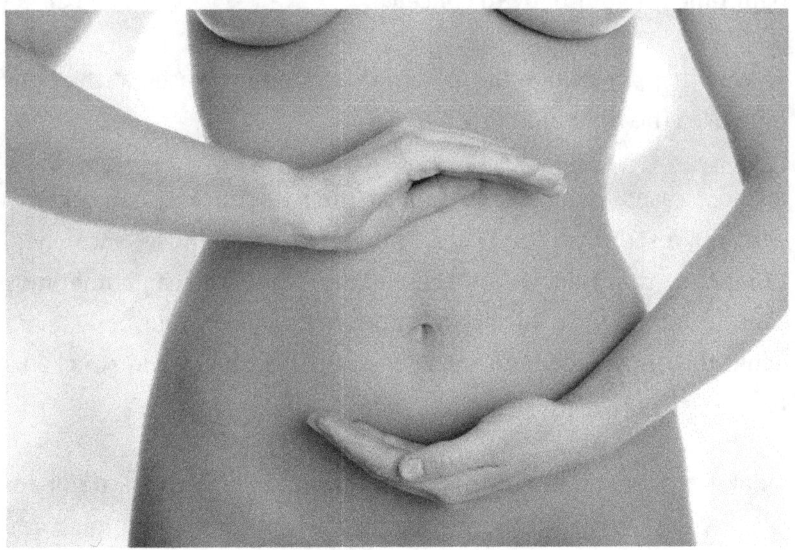

The human body is an amazingly complex thing. Biologically, we're designed to run efficiently by ingesting nutritious foods that give us the energy to exert ourselves physically, but also to fuel the neurons that fire within our brains.

Our brains are hundreds of times more complex than the most advanced computers on the planet. A brain is capable of keeping your body running on unconscious actions, such as breathing, or keeping your heart pumping, but it's also capable of releasing various hormones that help us to cope with everything we face during the day.

Your own body will release certain hormones to let you know its tired, different hormones when it's time to wake up, more hormones when you're feeling happy and different ones again when you're stressed or upset.

That's not even counting the myriad of hormones, enzymes and other goodies your brain releases to tell your body it's the optimum time to release an egg from one of your ovaries at the right time for your body to conceive.

So what happens when those hormones aren't released at the right time or in the right amounts?

In most cases, people tend to visit their doctor and come home with a prescription for drugs to help regulate those hormones. What they don't know is those chemical cocktails can sometimes cause other issues with the smooth functioning of your body, even while they might be addressing the initial problem you sought to fix.

Think for a moment about how your body might be a little like a car. If you put the wrong type of gasoline into your car's tank, it's not likely to run very well. If you put cooking oil instead of motor oil into the engine, it's very likely to break down completely.

Now think about what you put into your own tank each and every day to keep your motor running.

You might think you're eating enough food to sustain you on a daily basis, but really think about what nutritional value you're adding into those meals.

Once again, to use the car analogy, if you were to fill your car's gas tank with water, it would be full – but it won't be full of what it needs to run properly.

The same is true with your body.

In order to really function properly and really respond to any kind of infertility treatments, you need to overhaul your current nutritional plan.

Look at some ways you can cut out the processed foods and replace it with healthier options. Are there any ways you could increase the nutrients you consume by replacing a few simple things?

Of course, it's also worth looking at what else you're putting into your body's tank. Things like caffeine, nicotine, alcohol and drugs can also reduce your chances of conceiving naturally, as they affect the normal functions of your body.

There are plenty of ways to add more nutritional value to your diet each day, but it's still important to realize why you're doing it.

Fighting the Blues

Did you know that researchers have found a link between high stress levels in women and infertility? When women suffer from stress, they release testosterone into their systems.

This can make them seem more aggressive, more upset, more moody and definitely less able to cope with the pressures of life without reaching breaking point.

To counteract these stress hormones, women need to release oxytocin, which reduces stress levels and brings about a sense of being in a loving, nurturing life.

Learning to combat stress effectively can play an important role in reversing infertility, as too much testosterone in your system can reduce the chances of you releasing the right pregnancy hormones you need to fall pregnant.

Reducing and Eliminating Toxins

Think about the enormous number of chemicals, toxins and other poisons we're exposed to each and every day of our lives. Even the products we use to clean the environments in which we live are nothing more than harsh, harmful chemicals.

If you knew you were cleaning your shower or toilet with chemicals that could be affecting your fertility rate, would you change brands? Will another brand actually have the same types of chemicals in it?

What about the shampoo and conditioner you use? They might make your hair feel and smell lovely, but do you know what the chemicals inside those products are made from – or what else they're used for?

Have you ever wondered why we're taught to spit out toothpaste after we've brushed our teeth instead of just swallowing the minty-tasting foam?

There are so many simple, routine things we do each and every day that could potentially be increasing the level of toxins in your body.

Of course, there are some other types of toxins that aren't so noticeable. Things like mercury levels in some types of fish can also affect your body's optimal function.

Foods to Avoid When Trying to Conceive

If you're already having trouble conceiving, you should consider cutting down on certain foods, or eliminating them from your diet altogether.

It's a well-known fact that caffeine intake can reduce your fertility rate by up to 50%. While you might think this means cutting out that coffee each morning, it's important to realize how many other foods and beverages contain hidden amounts of caffeine that could be affecting your ovulation rate and your hormonal balances.

Things like chocolate and soda also contain caffeine. There are also some pain relievers that contain amounts of caffeine, such as Anacin and Excedrin. It's important to read labels if you're unsure of anything just to rule out those hidden sources of caffeine.

Alcohol is also detrimental to your fertility rate. Eliminate it from your diet by as much as four months before conceiving. The same is true for smoking.

Foods to Add to Your Diet When Trying to Conceive

It's been well-documented that foods that are low in fat and high in fiber will help to increase your body's overall health. Add simple things into your diet that include fruits, legumes, vegetables and nuts, as well as sensible choices for lean meat or chicken.

Finding foods that contain natural sources of folic acid and Vitamin B will also help to boost your natural immune system and help you to create a viable environment for conception to take place. Folic acid also helps to prevent birth defects, like spina bifida, and can also help reduce the incidence of miscarriage.

Some good natural sources of folic acid and vitamin B are green leafy vegetables, avocado, asparagus, papaya, broccoli, eggs, oranges, nuts, beans and wheat breads.

Oysters are also high on the list of foods to add to improve fertility, as they have a high zinc factor. It's well documented that males and females with zinc deficiencies may experience reduced fertility levels, so oysters can help.

Of course, just adding one or two types of foods to your diet might improve your chances of conceiving a little, but they won't cure infertility. A well-balanced diet, coupled with moderate exercise will help improve your overall health and hormonal levels.

Optimizing Your Health

When you improve your diet, your body is far more able to generate the right levels and types of hormones you need to feel good, be healthy and respond very well to infertility treatments.

You may also find that a relaxed 30 minute walk each day could increase your health even further. You'll be outside, which increases your Vitamin D intake and you'll be exercising moderately, which boosts your endorphin levels.

You may also find you begin to lose weight and have far more energy throughout the day.

There are plenty of health benefits to be had by eating the right kinds of foods with the correct levels of nutrition, vitamins and minerals, but the real importance is your own biological awareness.

You see, your brain may be choosing not to release the right hormones into your system in order for you to get pregnant naturally until it feels as though the right environment has been created to nurture an embryo to term.

What's more, it's been shown in several medical studies that improving your diet and lifestyle can actually reduce ovarian cysts and reduce menstrual cramps.

Of course, improving your diet and hormonal levels are only one aspect of beating infertility. There are plenty of other considerations to think about, too.

Chapter 3- The Common Misinformation about Sex and Infertility

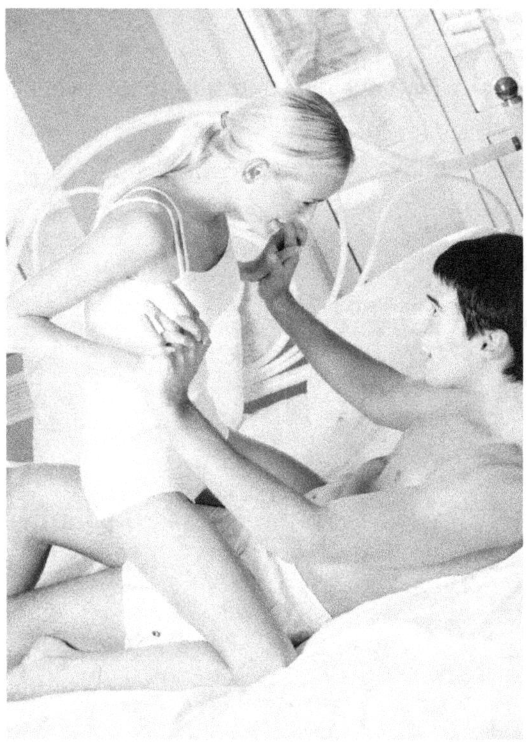

There is a lot of misinformation around about when you should have sex in order to improve your chances of conceiving. In schools, teenagers are taught that they could have sex at any time during their cycle and fall pregnant, but this is not accurate.

The best time to have sex in order to conceive is ideally 2-3 days before you ovulate. This is your most fertile time and you have the highest chances of conceiving before you actually release an egg.

Of course, this leads to the problem of knowing exactly when you're going to ovulate in the first place.

Ideally, a monthly menstrual cycle should last 28 days, with day one being the first day of your period. Some doctors state that ovulation is usually on day 14 of a menstrual cycle; so many women decide to plan to have sex on day 14, hoping to increase their chances of getting pregnant.

The problem with this approach is that not every woman has an exact 28 day cycle. Similarly, not every woman will ovulate on exactly day 14. You might ovulate on day 10 or on day 17.

There are ways to predict ovulation using basal body temperature kits or ovulation predictor kits, both of which are available at most pharmacies.

However, the single most reliable predictor of when you're at your most fertile point of the month is on the day you notice the most fertile cervical mucus discharge.

Cervical mucus is the discharge that is sticky, clear and a little like raw egg white. Having sex when you notice the cervical mucus is important, simply because this discharge is what aids sperm in surviving and swimming to the egg more effectively.

Timing When to Have Sex

Unfortunately, when many women decide to put off having sex until they notice their cervical mucus discharge, they tend to abstain completely until it's the "right time". They also tend to avoid sex at other times during the cycle.

This can mean sex becomes a chore or a routine. It becomes less about love and connection, which can increase strain on a relationship and increase stress levels for both of you.

Of course, you may also find that, even though the woman might be at her peak fertility time, you could be reducing the male's sperm quality without even knowing it.

You see, if you wait to have sex for a week or two before you notice the signs of ovulation, you risk your partner's sperm quality being at less than peak quality.

This is because a male's sperm quality and quantity will peak after only one or two days of abstinence. If you've made him wait for 10, the quality and quantity may not be ideal for optimum fertility rates.

Ideally, if you're planning to conceive, having sex twice a week, regardless of the fertility signs can actually strengthen the connection between you, as well as increase fertility for each of you at the same time.

Stop timing when to have sex and work on having a little fun together instead.

Good Sex = Better Chances of Conception

As mentioned in the previous section, many women become so preoccupied in trying to figure out the right time of the month to have sex that they forget about having fun and enjoying it.

When you have sex based on a calendar or a time table, it can lose a lot of the 'fun' factor. This can build resentment and cause stress, which can become a factor in keeping you infertile.

Researchers have shown that women who orgasm during sex can increase their chances of falling pregnant. This is because the spasmodic contractions of the uterus can actually help pull the sperm further into the uterus rather than remaining in the vagina where it can leak out far more easily.

Sex Positions

Yes, there are some sexual positions that are naturally going to help your chances of conception better than others. Of course, it's still possible to get pregnant with any position at all. However, some positions may help increase your chances.

Keep in mind that if a woman enjoys sex on top, this could reduce the chances of as much sperm getting to where it needs to go. Gravity plays a part here, so if you're on top, the sperm is going to leak out more easily.

For the more adventurous types, you might be a little disappointed to hear that missionary position is still the leading favorite position for optimal conception.

Ideally, place a pillow under your hips to tilt your pelvis up, but be sure the pillow isn't too large, as you don't want the sperm pooling behind your cervix. This will also help keep the sperm in longer and give the sperm more time to easily swim up through the cervix where it needs to go to reach the egg. Don't get up immediately after sex to wash or wipe, either. Allow the sperm to stay in for as long as possible.

However, if you have a tipped uterus, you may find that the "doggy position" might be more beneficial for you. Go ahead and get onto your hands and knees, and encourage your partner to enter from behind. He'll have fun and you'll be increasing your chances of getting that sperm where it needs to go.

There's still a lot of fun to be had experimenting with variations on the missionary position without reducing your conception odds. See what you and your partner can come up with to work on ways to add spice to the missionary position to increase the fun factor, while still remaining in the right position for the most possible sperm to reach your uterus.

Boy or Girl?

There is a preconception that having sex at a certain time or eating certain foods or having sex in a particular position might increase your chances of conceiving a boy or a girl.

While there are some suggestions that you can increase your chances of conceiving a baby of a particular sex during certain times of your ovulation period, these are not foolproof.

When you consider that a male will ejaculate millions of sperm upon orgasm, trying to aim at one specific type of these is going to be a hit and miss operation.

Basically, men produce two types of sperm: an X and a Y. The slower, larger X sperm will become female, while the faster, smaller Y sperm will be male.

This is where timing when you have sex becomes important.

Keep in mind there is no guaranteed way to determine the sex of your baby, but you can work on ways to favor your odds for or against one or the other.

Trying for a Girl

If you're trying for a girl, you will need to try and have sex seven days before ovulation and then every day until around 3 or more days prior to ovulation. Then try to avoid sex for a few days until you're sure ovulation is over.

This is because the smaller, faster Y sperm will reach the uterus and die before the egg is even released. However, there will still be a number of slower, larger X sperm alive when you ovulate.

Another theory is to work on shallower penetration. This has to do with the pH levels within the vagina. An acidic environment will kill the weaker Y sperm first, leaving a far greater quantity of X sperm remaining to fertilize the egg.

Besides, with deeper penetration, the sperm is deposited much closer to the egg, which can mean the faster Y sperm may reach their destination before the X sperm can.

You may also decrease the acidity levels within the vagina if you reach orgasm during sex. If you're trying for a girl, it may be best not to reach orgasm, as your body will release a substance that could make the vagina more alkaline instead of acidic.

Trying for a Boy

When trying for a boy, it may become important to try and not have sex until you reach around 2-3 days before ovulation. Then have sex every day until after ovulation has occurred.

Sex should involve deep penetration to deposit the sperm as close as possible to the cervix, and work towards having an orgasm during sex to pull even more sperm into the womb for better success.

It's also been noted that, while women should not drink any caffeine while drinking to conceive, one strong cup of coffee prior to sex for the MAN could actually increase the motility of the Y sperm, increasing your chances of having a boy.

Chapter 4- Getting Your Body Used to Carrying a Baby

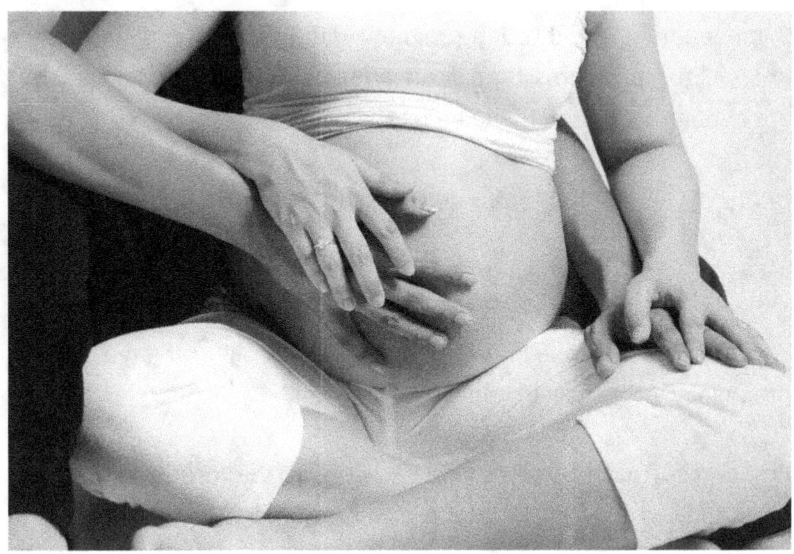

These are general descriptions, meant to give you an idea of what is normal and when you should be concerned.

As always, if you have a question or become concerned, you should contact your doctor.

In the sections that follow you will find guidelines for nutrition and exercise, and a lot of helpful information on the changes that occur during each trimester.

And you'll find out how to take care of your body and adjust your schedule and your life style during each stage of your pregnancy.

After you find out you are pregnant, after the excitement and buzz has worn off, you should expect the physical reality to set in.

During pregnancy you may experience fatigue, tenderness in your breasts, morning sickness, etc. Not every woman has every symptom.

Some women SAIL through pregnancy and others seem to endure lots of little problems that don't amount of anything serious, but are enough to disrupt life in general.

Here are some of the things you may encounter during pregnancy:

Fatigue

You may feel 'bone tired' or become easily fatigued during pregnancy, especially in your first trimester.

Remember that your body is working harder producing certain hormones and supplying blood and nutrients to your baby in the womb.

One of the hormones, progesterone, is a central nervous system depressant, so this hormone can make you feel drowsy or sleepy.

Try to pamper yourself during this time. Many women find that after their first trimester, they have renewed energy and stamina. In the meantime, take naps or just rest if you can.

Bleeding

It is not unusual to have a small amount of spotting or bleeding early in pregnancy – around 10 to 14 days after conception.

This bleeding is a bit earlier, spottier and 'pinker' in color than a usual menstrual cycle and it doesn't last very long.

Talk to your doctor and let him know about this, but don't be concerned unless the bleeding is heavy and lasts a long time. You may also get a bit of cramping early in pregnancy.

Changes in Appetite or Food Preferences

The smell of some foods may cause nausea during early pregnancy.

Or you may find you have a craving for certain foods during late pregnancy. The famous 'ice cream and pickles' legend is not so far from the truth for some women!

Many women find that they can no longer abide coffee during early pregnancy, and that this aversion subsides as their pregnancy progresses. Among the foods that may wreak havoc on your stomach: Meat, cheese or milk, and spicy foods. Don't be surprised if these preferences and aversions change as your pregnancy progresses.

Morning Sickness, Nausea and Vomiting

Usually, women experience these during early pregnancy, though some have this symptom for up to six months.

Most women encounter morning sickness for about a month during their first trimester, and symptoms can start as early as 14 days after conception.

Morning sickness is not always confined to the morning, and it results from the changing levels of estrogen in the body.

Some women experience morning sickness with no trigger, while others will become nauseous from certain smells like cigarette or cigar smoke, strong perfume, coffee or the smell of certain foods cooking.

Increased Urination

As your uterus enlarges, you are likely to feel the urge to go to the bathroom more often. This is normal during the first and third trimester.

Breast Tenderness and Changes

Increased production of the estrogen and progesterone is required to prepare the breasts for nursing.

During the early stages of pregnancy, some women complain that their breasts become so tender and sensitive that they can't even sleep on their stomach or touch the tissue on their breasts without discomfort.

This tenderness does pass. Women who are flat-chested often welcome the changes that pregnancy brings, as their breasts increase in size.

Be sure to buy and wear a comfortable bra, with plenty of support, during and after pregnancy to accommodate these changes. If you are planning to nurse your baby, you will want to look for special 'nursing bras' to make nursing easier.

Headaches

Many pregnant women complain of mild headaches that occur frequently, early in pregnancy. These headaches occur because of increased blood circulation caused by hormonal fluctuation and changes in the body.

Constipation and Bloating

Constipation is common during early pregnancy because of an increase in progesterone that slows digestion. Drink plenty of water to keep your body hydrated and help ease constipation and bloating.

Mood Fluctuation

Again, it is all due to the hormonal changes in your body. You may be an even-tempered person and suddenly find yourself crying or losing your temper for no reason.

Understand that these mood swings are common during the first trimester and will usually improve.

Dizziness

Early in your pregnancy you may feel dizzy or faint because of low blood sugar and changes in circulation and hormone levels.

Be sure to drink plenty of water and keep crackers and other healthy snacks on hand to address low blood sugar and don't be surprised if you need to rest and pamper yourself a bit more, especially during early pregnancy.

Weight Gain and Changes in Center of Gravity

Your balance and center of gravity are going to change as your body changes.

Don't try to walk a tightrope or a ladder in your new, 'enhanced' condition!

Wear sensible shoes without high heels so you can balance and walk more easily without falling or stumbling.

Most mothers gain 25 to 35 pounds, some as much as 50-60 pounds during pregnancy.

And that additional can make you uncomfortable, causing back strain and soreness. 50% of all pregnant women develop low-back pain at some time during their pregnancy.

Be sure to use your legs when you are lifting and use common sense when lifting or climbing during pregnancy.

Increased and displaced weight puts more stress on joints and as the baby grows, your lower back must compensate for this weight.

We'll talk about exercise in a little while, but for now, understand that it is important to keep your muscles strong and limber during this time, in order to avoid back strain and fatigue.

Chapter 5- The Importance of Good Health for You and Your Unborn Child

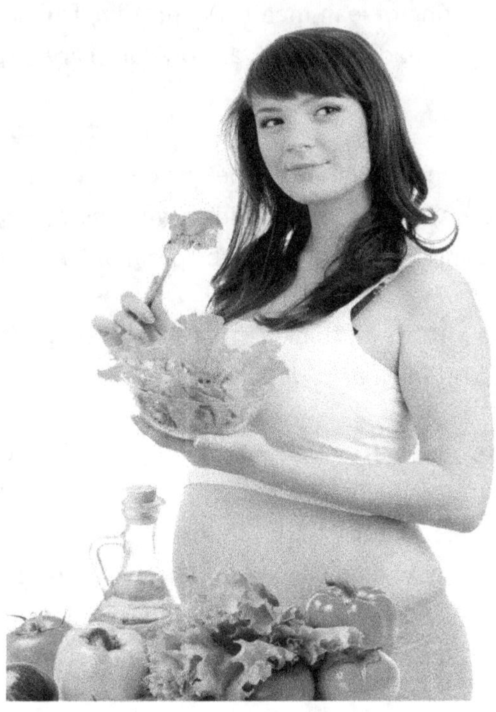

Now that you are pregnant, it is no time to diet. You certainly want to eat the right things and try not to gain an unhealthy amount of weight, but you should NOT be dieting right now.

- You will need about 300 to 350 calories more per day than when you were eating just for you – about 2,500 to 2,700 calories per day.

- If you are very thin by nature or if you are going through a multiple birth pregnancy, your doctor may even prescribe more of an increase in daily caloric intake.

- On the other hand, if you are typically overweight, your doctor may advise that you consume more calories, but she may advise you to drop below the additional 300 to 350 usually prescribed for an average pregnancy.

You should plan to maintain a well-balanced diet throughout your pregnancy, consisting of lean meats and protein, fruits, vegetables, and whole-grain breads, as well as low-fat dairy products like cheese and milk.

Your doctor will probably prescribe prenatal vitamins for you. These are special vitamins compounded with the correct amounts of calcium, iron and folic acid needed by pregnant women.

Don't make the mistake of thinking that your prenatal vitamins will cover all the nutritional needs you have.

You still need to eat well!

We have provided details here, so that you can build a good nutritional base for your own health, and for the health of your unborn child. As always, if you have any questions throughout the course of your pregnancy, please consult your doctor.

Let's look at the details of your nutritional building blocks:

Vegetables and Fruits

You should have 4 or more servings of vegetables and 3 or more servings of fruits, at minimum.

Here are some examples of serving sizes:

Fruits: One medium-sized apple or banana, one half cup of chopped fruit or three quarters of a cup of fruit juice.

Vegetables: One cup of leafy vegetable (raw), one half cup of non-leafy vegetable (either cooked or raw) or three quarters of a cup of a vegetable juice (like tomato juice)

Eating fruits and vegetables that contain Vitamin C will help you absorb iron, heal minor wounds and maintain healthy gums and body tissue. Examples of these types of vegetables and fruits include:

Fruits: Papaya, tomato, orange, melon, strawberry

Vegetables: Peppers, cabbage, broccoli, green leafy vegetables like spinach and escarole.

Protein

Strive to have two or more servings of lean, cooked meat or poultry (without the skin), or fish. These servings should amount to 60 grams of protein per day.

Here are some examples of serving sizes:

Meat, Poultry, Fish:

Strive for two to three ounces of cooked meat, poultry or fish. Do NOT eat undercooked or UNCOOKED meat, poultry or fish. These may contain bacteria and can make you very sick! Avoid 'lunch meat', 'cold cuts' or 'deli meats'.

Try to stay away from fish with high mercury content (shark, swordfish, tilefish (white snapper or golden snapper) and king mackerel.

These fish tend to contain more mercury content, which can be harmful to your baby. Do not eat more than six ounces of tuna or tuna steak per week.

Other Proteins: One third cup of nuts, 1 cooked egg, one half cup of tofu or cooked beans or peas, or two tablespoons of peanut butter.

Eating protein helps you to build muscle, and keeps you healthy and strong. It also helps your body to provide antibodies for your baby. Protein contains the B Vitamins and iron important to produce rich, red blood cells and keep your blood strong.

Protein is especially important during your second and third trimester, as it will help your body keep up with the demands and growth of your baby in the womb.

Whole Grains and Whole Grain Products

Have at least nine or more servings of whole grain products per day. Try to stay away from white flour, sweetened cereals, etc. They contain little or no nutritional value.

Here are some examples of serving sizes:

Whole Wheat or Other Whole Grain Bread: One slice

Cooked (hot) Cereal, Brown Rice or Whole Grain Pasta: One half cup

Cold Cereal: One cup

These products contain B Vitamins, and minerals and fiber to keep your body healthy and keep your digestive system moving.

Folic acid is often added to cold breakfast cereals and to 'enriched' grain products and this is also an important mineral for your body during pregnancy. Look at the packaging and try to choose products that contain more folic acid, wherever possible.

Dairy Products

Have four or more servings per day. While you are pregnant, you will want to consume about at least 1,000 mg (milligrams) of calcium per day (1,300 milligrams if you are under eighteen years of age).

If you cannot get that much calcium in your diet, ask your doctor about your prenatal vitamins to be sure that you are getting enough calcium by looking at your combined diet and supplements.

If you find that you are lactose intolerant, you can use reduced lactose products, or take tablets to increase your tolerance of dairy products. Talk to your doctor to find out which solution will work best for you.

Here are some examples of serving sizes of dairy products:

Cheese (natural, not processed): One and one half ounces

Low-Fat or Non-Fat Milk: One cup

Natural (active ingredient) Yogurt: One cup

Conceive a Baby Naturally

You and your growing baby both need lots of calcium to keep your bones and your teeth strong. Dairy products contain Vitamins A and D, and also protein, and B Vitamins. Vitamin A is important for your baby's growth, and for immune system support.

Water

6-8 eight ounce glasses of water per day (if you are exercising: 8-10 glasses)

This may seem like a lot but your body will adjust to this volume, and you need to stay hydrated during pregnancy to prevent constipation, hemorrhoids, swelling, dehydration, urinary and bladder infections, and muscle strain.

Vitamins and Minerals

We've talked about how important it is to follow a good diet during pregnancy. Your prenatal vitamins, combined with the good food you eat should give you enough of the right vitamins and minerals.

If you look at the label of your prenatal vitamin bottle, you should see plenty of the following vitamins and minerals.

Calcium

Most women don't get enough calcium (1,000 mg per day) but when you are pregnant your need for calcium is even more important, to meet the demands of your body and the demands of your baby's calcium needs to grow strong bones.

Be sure your prenatal vitamins contain 1,000 mg (1,300 if you are under eighteen) per dose.

Iron

You need iron to produce hemoglobin and red blood cells. Hemoglobin is the component of red blood cells that carries oxygen throughout your system.

It supplies all your cells and your baby's body and organs with plenty of rich oxygenated blood with which to grow and remain healthy.

Your body and your baby's body also need iron to grow bones and teeth and to prevent anemia. Be sure your prenatal vitamins contain 27 to 30 mg of iron per dose.

Folic Acid (Folate)

Studies show that taking folic acid supplements during pregnancy decreases the risk of neural tube defects by up to 70%!

The neural tube contains your baby's spinal cord and developing brain, and when it does not form properly it can cause serious conditions like spina bifida, and congenital heart disease.

Because your body uses folic acid very early in pregnancy, it is wise to start taking a supplement if you are planning a pregnancy.

Check your prenatal vitamins to be sure you are getting 400 micrograms (0.4 milligrams) per dose.

Pregnancy and Diabetes

If you are a diabetic and you want to get pregnant, work with your OB/GYN doctor and your diabetes doctor to be sure you are in the best shape possible at least three to six months before you conceive.

Then be sure you are followed regularly by both physicians so that you remain healthy during your pregnancy and after delivery.

During your pregnancy you should monitor your diet and exercise program and look for signs of imbalance in your blood sugar, as pregnancy can sometimes wreak havoc on your regular routine and your insulin levels.

You may have to get a special meal plan from a nutritionist or dietician in order to compensate for the changes in your body and your blood sugar and ensure that your child does not experience problems or birth defects because of high blood sugar levels that may cross into the placenta.

Talk to your doctor about getting more B Vitamins, especially folic acid to guard against the risk of birth defects.

If you have never been diabetic in the past, you may find yourself facing 'gestational diabetes', which is a form of diabetes that occurs during pregnancy and typically disappears after delivery.

This form of diabetes is usually controlled with diet, medication, and exercise, but it must be treated in order to ensure that you and your baby remain healthy.

Your OB/GYN doctor will usually refer you to a dietitian so you can get meal plans that are specially designed to help you control your blood sugar.

Vegetarian Diets

If you are a strict 'vegan' and eat no animal products or animal byproducts, you may feel you will have a problem during pregnancy. Or perhaps you are a 'lacto-ovo-vegan' and you do eat eggs and dairy products.

If you wish to maintain a vegan diet during pregnancy, by all means you should find a doctor who is willing to support this approach and stay in close contact with her regarding your nutritional health and your baby's health, as your pregnancy progresses.

Here are some nutritional guidelines that will help you stay healthy and deliver a healthy baby.

To get all the protein and calcium you need – the biggest problem faced by most vegans – you will want to eat appropriate amounts of the following things:

• dried peas (split peas are great),

• dried beans (cooked) including navy beans, kidney or red beans, black or lima beans and white beans,

• Soy products like tempeh, tofu and tofu cheese,

• Almonds and other nuts, and butter made from nut oils,

• Soy milk or goat milk or cow milk (if you drink it), and/or

• Active yogurt

• Turnip greens,

• Oranges,

• Broccoli,

• Molasses,

• fortified cereals,

• Wheat germ,

• Spinach,

• Raisins

The great thing about a vegetarian diet is that it is already high in folic acid and B Vitamins and that is important to your baby's health and growth.

However, you may find it hard to get your extra 300-350 calories per day if you are eating a vegetarian diet.

Your diet, while high in fiber, with plenty of vegetables, fruits and grains, tends to be low in calories and you don't feel hungry enough to eat more because all that fiber will fill you up!

Talk to your doctor about this, if you find that it is a problem. You may want to take a caloric supplement.

Things You Should Avoid in Your Diet

What you DON'T eat or drink during your pregnancy can be just as important as what you DO consume!

Here are some things to avoid while you are pregnant:

Alcohol

We shouldn't have to tell you this, but we will anyway! STAY AWAY FROM ALCOHOL DURING PREGNANCY.

A glass of wine or bottle of beer may seem harmless enough but no study has yet to determine how much is a safe amount of alcohol and how much can cause mental retardation, central nervous system damage, brain damage, and birth defects in your baby.

It is better to be safe than sorry!

Alcohol goes straight into your baby's body in high concentration levels through your blood stream, through the umbilical cord and into the placenta, and can cause any one of an array of symptoms included in Fetal Alcohol Spectrum Disorder (FASD).

Children with FASD can have learning disabilities, memory and attention disorders, as well as language, and vision, or hearing problems, to name a few. So save that glass of wine or bottle of beer and enjoy it after you delivery your healthy child!

Caffeine

Consuming a lot of caffeine can increase your chance of miscarriage. Two or three cups a day may not seem like much to you, but just to be safe, you should try to stop drinking coffee altogether.

If you find you cannot do so, at least try to cut it down to one cup per day or start drinking decaffeinated coffee!

And remember that there are other beverages and foods that contain high concentrations of caffeine. Green tea and black tea, cola sodas (pop), even chocolate.

You can have these things in moderation (one cup of tea or a half of glass of soda or a candy bar once a week), because the caffeine content in these products is typically much less than that contained in cup of coffee (90-140 mg of caffeine).

You'll be happy to know that the average candy bar only contains 5-30 mg of caffeine, but you still need to consider the FAT content in that candy and remember the word: MODERATION

Foods to Avoid

Avoid foods that MAY carry bacteria and other food-borne illness (toxoplasmosis and listeriosis to name two). These can cause birth defects and miscarriage, and while you may be able to eat them with no problems, you may not want to take the risk during your pregnancy.

- Un-pasteurized (soft) cheeses, often labeled as 'fresh cheese' like feta cheese, goat cheese, brie, camembert, and blue or limburger cheeses.

- Un-pasteurized milk, juice, or apple cider

- Raw eggs or foods that contain raw eggs like tiramisu, mousse, cookie or cake batter, homemade ice cream, Caesar dressing (if made fresh).

- Raw fish like sushi and CERTAINLY raw meat

- High mercury content fish like shark, swordfish, tilefish (white snapper or golden snapper), and king mackerel

If you are a health advocate and you routinely take herbs, please do NOT take these particular herbs while you are pregnant:

- Arbor vitae
- Autumn crocus
- Barberry
- Basil oil
- Beth root
- Black cohosh
- Bloodroot
- Blue cohosh
- Broom
- Bugleweed
- Clove oil
- Comfrey
- Cotton root
- Devil's claw
- Dong quai
- False unicorn root
- Feverfew
- Golden seal
- Greater celandine
- Juniper and juniper oil
- Lady's mantle
- Liferoot
- Mistletoe
- Mugwort (avoid during pregnancy & breast feeding)
- American pennyroyal
- European pennyroyal (avoid during pregnancy & breast feeding)

- Peruvian bark
- Pokeroot
- Pseudo ginseng
- Pulsatilla (limit use while breast feeding)
- Rue
- Sassafras
- Shepherd's purse
- Southernwood (avoid during pregnancy & breast feeding)
- Squill
- Tansy
- Wild yam
- Wormwood (avoid during pregnancy & breast feeding)

Chapter 6 - Keep Your Strength through Exercise

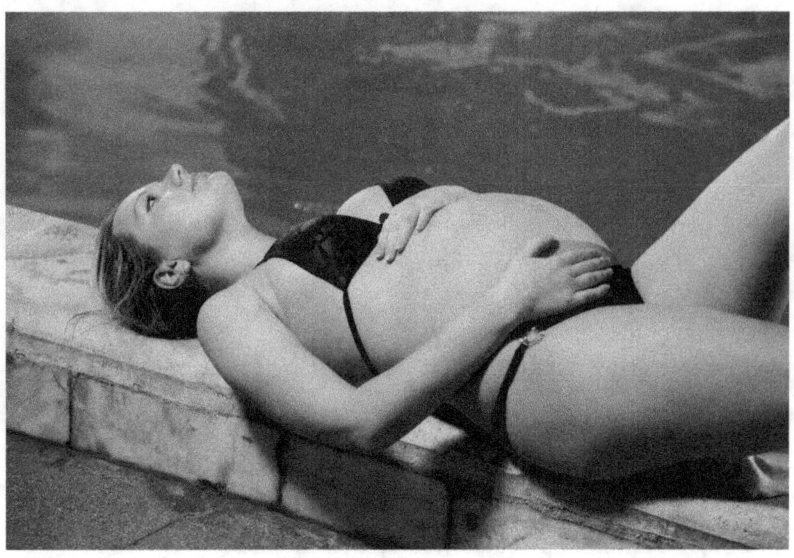

Unless you have a serious problem or abnormality in your pregnancy, you should expect to continue to exercise throughout your term.

If you have NOT exercised in the past, you will, of course, want to consult your doctor to determine the level and frequency of exercise you can do during your pregnancy.

Exercise during pregnancy is healthy and will help to reduce swelling and bloat, prevent excessive weight gain, reduce muscle and back strain, and constipation, improves your energy levels, your sleep patterns and your mood.

It will also help you stay in shape for labor and reduce your recovery time after delivery.

Conceive a Baby Naturally

The best kind of exercise during pregnancy is exercise with moderate strain and intensity (brisk walking, and swimming are great choices).

There are also yoga and Pilates classes designed specifically for pregnant women to provide them with strength conditioning, and flexibility.

Many of these classes are available on video and DVD so look in your local book store or online.

Meditation and relaxation classes are also great to relieve work, family and pregnancy related stress and to prepare you mentally and emotionally for the delivery marathon.

Remaining calm and relaxed can ease your delivery tremendously and these techniques should not be overlooked.

Remember that it is just as important to exercise and prepare your brain as it is to exercise your body!

Avoid exercise like high-impact aerobics, rock climbing, gymnastics that require balance or exercise at high elevations. Don't water ski, snow ski or ride a horse and use common sense when exercising during pregnancy.

Always ask your doctor before undertaking or pursuing an exercise program.

You should also know that among the hormones your body will adjust during your pregnancy is one that may make you more prone to muscle pulls and strain.

Since your body is preparing for delivery, this hormone will loosen and relax certain ligaments and muscles, and make you more prone to injury when doing certain kinds of exercise that require balance or lifting.

Keep this in mind when you go on vacation and participate in activities you don't usually try, when you exercise, or even when you lift your toddler nephew.

You may find that your knees, legs, back and pelvis are more sensitive to strain and injury, especially during late pregnancy.

Stretch before exercise to get your muscles warmed up so you are less likely to strain them.

When you are exercising take plenty of breaks and drink a lot of water to keep you hydrated.

Try to exercise for 30 minutes, three times per week if you can.

Swimming is a great way to work out because you will be buoyant and feel light as a feather in the water, and there is no strain or jerking involved in this exercise.

Walking is also great exercise and it does not jar your joints or shins as much as jogging.

Even women, who have not exercised before pregnancy, can usually begin a regimen of walking and work up to 30 minutes, three times a week on a gradual schedule.

IF you were a jogger before pregnancy, you may be able to continue this activity with some modification to schedule and intensity.

Talk to your doctor about it.

Wear good shoes and watch your balance. Remember your center of gravity has changed so you may be more prone to falls on uneven surfaces while walking or jogging.

Monitor your pulse and be sure that your heart rate does not exceed 140 beats per minute.

Do not participate in strenuous activity for more than 15 minutes at a time.

If you feel tired, overheated or dizzy, or if you get nauseous, weak or have blurred vision or heart palpitations, stop immediately and sit down and rest.

If these feelings do not pass within a few minutes after stopping the activity, call your doctor immediately.

Chapter 7 - Do You Need to Change Your Lifestyle for Your Growing Baby?

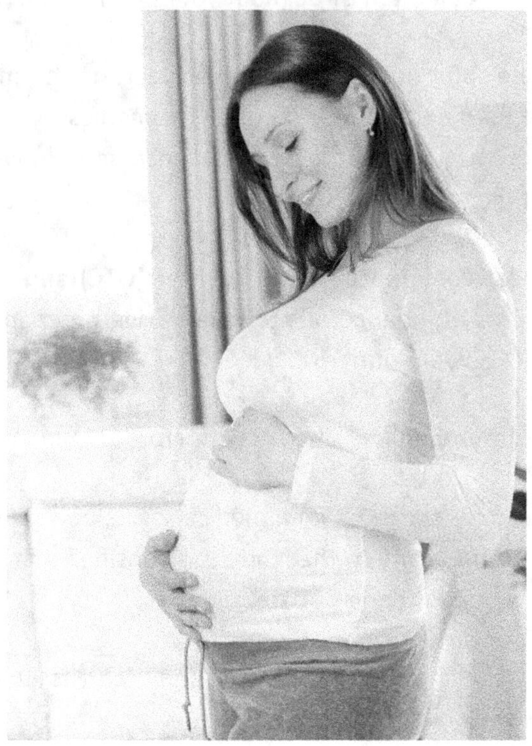

Food and exercise are important components of a healthy pregnancy; so is the way you live your life.

Your lifestyle considerations include everything from the medications you take, and the amount of sleep you get, to the level of stress you experience on a daily basis.

Let's look at some of the factors you need to consider in your lifestyle:

Medication, Drugs and Medical Treatment

If you are taking prescription or over the counter medication, talk to your OB/GYN doctor about these medications and be sure you can continue taking them throughout your pregnancy.

There may be safer options you can consider, or you may have to stop taking medications, natural remedies, vitamins or supplements that are not absolutely necessary to your health during this time.

Even the most common over the counter (OTC) and prescription medications may be dangerous to take during pregnancy because of their effect on your unborn child.

Don't make assumptions. Talk to your doctor!

If you are seeing a specialist for a medical issue, be sure to let them know you are pregnant so that they can consider that and talk to your OB/GYN doctor if appropriate.

Remember to tell x-ray technicians and dentists that you are pregnant as well.

Ask your doctor to give you a list of 'safe over the counter medications' for things like muscle strain and headache, so you will know what to take if you need pain medication, allergy medication, etc.

As to illegal or narcotic drugs, if you are pregnant and you taking these drugs (once or frequently) you are placing your baby at risk for premature birth, birth defect, miscarriage, learning disability and lots of other things.

If you are addicted to a drug your baby can also be born addicted. Talk to your doctor about this and get help immediately.

There is no time to waste!

If you have used drugs at any time during your pregnancy, tell your doctor. Even if you stopped using the drug or didn't know you were pregnant when you used it, your baby can still be a risk and your doctor may need to monitor your pregnancy more closely.

Smoking

If you smoke and you are pregnant, get help and quit. There is no other way to say it!

Pregnant women who smoke reduce the circulation to their own bodies and to their baby, and they pass nicotine and carbon monoxide through the placenta and into the baby's body.

The risks of smoking are legendary and they have significant impact on your pregnancy, including:

• Premature birth

• Stillborn fetus

• Low birth weight stillbirth

• Sudden infant death syndrome (SIDS)

• Asthma and upper respiratory problems

Do what you have to do to quit NOW!

Sleep

You are going to need more sleep during your pregnancy and you should plan for that. Don't try to stay up until midnight to get that report done. Just give in to the fatigue and allow yourself more rest, especially during your first trimester when you are likely to feel 'bone tired'.

As your baby grows it may become difficult to find a comfortable sleep position. Most doctors recommend lying on your side with your knees bent and putting a pillow between your knees to take the strain off your lower back.

Lying on your side also makes things easier on your heart and lungs, and the baby's weight and size will not be so likely to put pressure on your blood vessels, so your legs are less likely to swell.

Sleeping on your side also helps to reduce the likelihood of varicose veins, constipation and hemorrhoids because it allows for better circulation and provide optimum blood flow to your baby and the placenta.

If you sleep on your LEFT SIDE, you are also relieving the pressure the baby's weight can put on your liver and improving blood supply to your kidneys so they can flush toxins out of your system.

Buy a few extra pillows and use them behind your back and under your stomach to give you more support.

Most stores carry full length 'body pillows', and even pregnancy pillows that are designed to support your body and your stomach.

Support and Ergonomics

If you sit a lot at work or during a commute or in a classroom, pay attention to the support you have for your back and legs during this time.

You will be sore and tired if your body is not supported appropriately.

Position your computer monitor so that the top of the screen is at or below your natural 'eye level' and elevate your feet on a stool, wastebasket or chair when you can.

Take a break every 30 minutes and walk around the office or down the hall to ask your co-worker a question. Keep moving to reduce swelling in your legs, ankles and feet and pain in your lower back.

Stress

Stress is a fact of life and it is unhealthy for everyone, but it is especially hard on you when you are pregnant and it is hard on your baby.

If your job, school or family life is stressful, if your schedule is crazy or if you are under a lot of pressure, you need to look for ways to reduce the stress.

You may have to stop working sooner if you can't find solutions at work. If your stress comes from a long or intense commute to work, consider ways to change that commute by working at home a few days a week.

Talk to your employer and your co-workers and enlist their help during the time you are pregnant. You can return the favor after you deliver.

Let your family help you with things you can afford to delegate and allow yourself to be pampered. Be willing to let things go. You don't have to vacuum every day. You can buy good takeout food on occasion and ask your husband to do the laundry.

Reduce the hours you work or study and try to get more relaxation time and rest time in your schedule.

You will be better prepared for a healthy delivery if you look seriously at this issue.

Taking Care of Your Cat

This is a great time to avoid cat litter. Pregnant women should NOT clean litter boxes, because of the risk of toxoplasmosis, spread through dirty cat litter.

Your baby may be born prematurely, suffer from poor growth or even have eye or brain damage if you are exposed to this toxic substance.

What makes this problem more serious is that you are likely to be symptom-free, while having passed toxoplasmosis to your child who child can then suffer from the effects of the toxin.

Watching Your Weight

You should (and will) gain weight during your pregnancy. Most of your weight gain will be during your third trimester. It is important to eat a balanced diet and exercise so that you do not gain excess weight that may hamper your recovery or your physical activity during or after pregnancy.

In general, your doctor will strive to limit your weight gain to:

• 2-4 pounds total during the first trimester

• 3-4 pounds per month during the second and third trimesters

• 25-30 pounds for an average total weight gain during pregnancy*

*if you were underweight before pregnancy: 28-40 pounds total weight gain, if you were overweight before pregnancy: 15-25 pounds total weight gain

Your total weight gain during pregnancy averages 6-8 pounds in 'baby weight', with the rest consisting of water retention, amniotic fluid, placental sac, and increased breast and uterine weight.

Of course everyone is different and weight gain depends on your personal situation, your height and your starting weight, as well. Talk to your doctor about what is right for you.

Studies have shown that women who gain more than the total recommended during pregnancy, and who do not lose this weight within six months after birth are at high risk for obesity as long as ten years after delivery.

Your doctor will monitor your weight gain at every visit and talk to you about any concerns he may have in that regard.

Sex during Pregnancy

Sex and pregnancy go hand in hand. But many pregnant women often have questions about sex DURING pregnancy. And sometimes pregnant women are embarrassed to ask their doctor questions about this intimate subject.

You may be concerned about whether intercourse can cause miscarriage or pose a risk to your unborn child.

Presuming you have a normal pregnancy, there is no fear of complications or problems resulting from sexual intercourse during pregnancy.

Of course you should ask your doctor about your own situation, but the average woman can and will have sex well into her third trimester.

If you start to get uncomfortable in your third trimester and it is difficult for you to achieve or sustain certain positions because of your physical size, you and your partner may want to experiment with pillows for support, or try new positions to make you more comfortable.

We don't recommend sex 'toys' during pregnancy because you don't want to introduce anything foreign that may have germs or bacteria on the surface.

Talk to your doctor about your concerns and, if you want to do some research, take a look online to find out more information and answer your specific questions.

Monica Libinski

From your first week of pregnancy to your last week of pregnancy you should consider and attend to your diet, your exercise and physical activity and lifestyle issues.

You may find it necessary to be more cautious and cease certain activities like skydiving, but in general, your pregnancy is a time when you will feel excited, healthy and NORMAL, in that you can do most anything you could do before you were pregnant.

Remember to take good care of your health so that your baby is born healthy and your delivery goes smoothly.

Most women say they feel healthy, well and happy during pregnancy. While they may experience some discomfort as they progress through the stages of pregnancy, they are far from being invalid, and do not wish to sit in bed, or hide in the back room as their great grandmothers might have done.

CHAPTER 8- WHAT TO EXPECT FROM THE FIRST TO THE LAST TRIMESTER

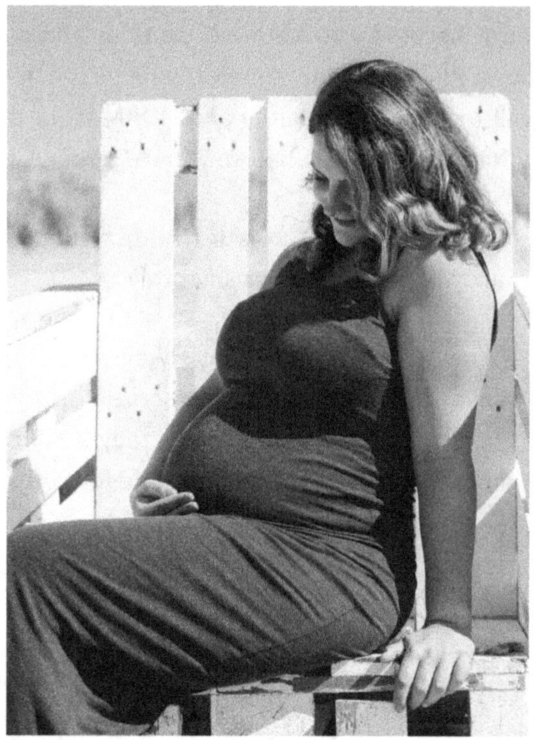

Now let's look at the three stages of pregnancy and talk about how your baby develops and how your body changes during these phases so you will know how to take care of yourself and your unborn child as your pregnancy progresses.

The First Trimester

If you don't already have an OB/GYN or if you want to find another health care professional, like a midwife to follow your pregnancy, you will need to start looking for a health care provider as soon as you think you are pregnant.

Monica Libinski

Finding the best obstetrician, family doctor or nurse/midwife can be a challenge. You may wish to ask friends with children and get some personal references you trust.

Make a list of the numbers you want to call and make an appointment for a consultation so you can meet the person before you decide.

Write down the questions you want to ask and make your own decisions.

Even though references are great, you may have a different set of expectations than your neighbor.

shining armor" when things went wrong during her labor without being fully aware that her doctor's interventions, such as inducing her labor too early, may have contributed to her birthing problems in the first place).

Check with the La Leche League by calling the listing in the white pages, or looking online at www.lalecheleague.org. They talk to pregnant and nursing women all the time and they know the local providers well.

Talk to at least three doctors or health care professionals so you know that you are choosing the one best for your style and preferences.

During the interview, ask if your health insurance will cover his/her care, ask about their experience and history delivering babies, and especially about experience with medical complications.

What hospitals or birthing centers do they attend? How often will you see them for visits and what kinds of tests will they do? How many C-sections do they perform vs. natural births? How can you reach them if you have a question or problem in between visits?

Once you have chosen your doctor or other health care professional, she/he will exam you and give you an estimated due date.

This exam may/will include blood and urine samples, a Pap smear and tests for HIV, syphilis, gonorrhea and chlamydia.

Remember that we said that your doctor will start your 'pregnancy clock' on the first day of your last menstrual cycle? You might be interested to know that the average pregnancy is 266 in length (38 weeks, not 40 weeks as calculated by your doctor).

The reason for this discrepancy is so that your doctor can take into consideration all the variables (stress, diet, variable menstrual cycles and other things).

Your doctor will give you an 'estimated due date' but if you want to figure it out for yourself you can use this calculation:

First, add 7days to the first day of your last menstrual period, then count forward 9 months. If your typical menstrual cycle is shorter or longer than 28 days, you will have to add or subtract more days to the 9 months to make the final estimated due date more accurate.

If you can't remember when your last menstrual period started, your doctor may suggest a sonogram to determine a more reasonable estimated due date, though this is not necessarily a precise way to calculate.

Monica Libinski

The fact is that when your baby is ready to be born, he/she will let you know!

A sonogram at any time during the first four months of your pregnancy can help your care provider establish your due date with a reasonable amount of accuracy, but babies' growth rates become more individual as they mature, and sonograms later on in pregnancy may not be as precise.

Less than 5% of babies arrive on the day they were predicted, so don't plan things around that day!

About one in five pregnancies results in a miscarriage, and this usually happens before the heart beat is detected. About one in eight babies arrives prematurely.

Unless there are health risks involved in a prolonged pregnancy or the bay seems to be jeopardy, your doctor will rarely suggest inducing labor. The best idea is to wait until the baby is ready.

Now that you understand your estimated due date, you will want to be sure you have all the information you need in between visits. Talk to your doctor about your diet, exercise and any medical family history you think is pertinent.

Go home! Eat right, take your prenatal vitamins, exercise and make any lifestyle changes you need to make.

If you have morning sickness, it should peak around the 8th week of your pregnancy.

Some women have more severe nausea than others, and up to 50% of pregnant women still have symptoms in their 20th week.

Other symptoms you will probably experience in your first trimester include fatigue and tenderness in your breasts.

In order to remember the things you want to discuss with your doctor at the next visit and to track dates, you may want to keep a 'pregnancy journal' and include your trimester milestones, when your next doctor's appointment is, what you have been eating and when you experienced any symptoms you want to discuss with your doctor.

If your questions are not urgent, write them down so you don't forget to ask the next time you see the doctor. If your questions or concerns are urgent, call your doctor right away.

At the end of your first trimester, your doctor may suggest a blood serum screening to determine your risk of having a baby with Down syndrome, open neural tube defect, or trisomy 18. She may also suggest a chorionic villus sampling if you have a family history of genetic problems. If your doctor suggests other tests, ask him why he is recommending these tests and what the results will tell him.

If test results are not good, remember that your doctor has more options and remedies for problem pregnancies than ever before in history. Get all the information about the issue and remain calm. Your doctor may suggest you see a specialist if her concerns are serious.

Pregnancy-related headaches can come from hormonal changes, dehydration and lots of other sources. If you experience a migraine headache during pregnancy, know that about 15% of pregnant women get migraines during this time, and it is usually during early pregnancy.

About 10-30 minutes before onset of a migraine, you may start to feel tired and nauseated. You may even get blurred vision or see tiny points of flashing light. Other symptoms can include a tingling sensation in your hands or legs and sensitivity to light and sound.

Ask your doctor how to treat these headaches and understand that they usually go away as your pregnancy progresses.

If your headache includes any of the following symptoms, call your doctor immediately: sudden or explosive head pain, headache accompanied by fever and/or stiff neck, headaches accompanied by slurred speech or serious vision problems.

If you work in a strenuous job or in a risky environment, you should tell your employer about your pregnancy immediately and talk to your doctor about taking your leave sooner or see if you can work in another section of the company temporarily.

An example of a risky job might be a job where you have to climb or balance (like a telephone repair job), a chemist, x-ray technician, medical disease research, or a job where you have to do a lot of lifting, or a job where you work in a poorly ventilated location, or where it is very hot or very cold all the time.

You should also be wary of jobs that require you to travel to countries where you might be exposed to exotic or contagious diseases.

The Second Trimester

During your second trimester you may still be experiencing morning sickness and you may have started to have headaches and a sensitivity and aversion to certain smells and foods.

If you have waited to tell your family, co-workers and friends about your pregnancy, you can probably do so now. Most women are skittish about announcing a pregnancy before the second trimester begins because miscarriage most often occurs during the first trimester.

If your appearance or your symptoms changed early in your pregnancy, you may already have been faced with this announcement.

If you work in a risky job or a strenuous or dangerous position, you have probably already told your employer you are pregnancy and decided on what you will do to protect your child and yourself during your pregnancy. If you have NOT done this, you need to do it ASAP.

During this trimester you will want to start thinking about and talking to your doctor about delivery-related issues.

Give yourself plenty of time to talk about these things and decide so you are not caught short when you are trying to prepare your home and family for the impending delivery during your first trimester.

Where will you have the baby, who will you choose as your pediatrician? Will you take childbirth classes and have a natural delivery or do you want to opt for pain medication during birth.

If you are going to take a childbirth course, ask your doctor for recommendations and remember that you will usually need a partner.

Another question you might discuss with your doctor is whether to breast feed or use formula?

Monica Libinski

As long as we are on the topic of breast feeding, let's talk about the changes in your breasts and how to best care for your breasts during pregnancy and prepare them for breast feeding, if that is your choice.

Your breasts are going to get bigger over the course of your pregnancy, and your rib cage will get wider to accommodate your growing baby.

You may notice tiny blue blood vessels on your chest as your blood vessels dilate and enlarge. Your nipples and areola (the dark area surrounding the nipple) will get larger and darker so that your newborn infant can more easily see them for nursing after birth.

Little bump may appear around your areola. These are oil glands that help to keep the area around your nipples clean for nursing.

Sometime around your 14th week of pregnancy, your nipples will start to leak a whitish fluid called 'colostrum'; a rich protein-filled form of early milk that will clear your child's digestive tract after delivery.

You can buy disposable breast to absorb leaks and keep your skin from getting irritated. Tuck them inside your bra and avoid embarrassing leaks!

Be sure you purchase a roomier bra to accommodate your enlarged breasts. You can consider wearing a nursing bra if you'd like. They are comfortable and have a lot of cushioning and stretch. To take care of your breasts as they change, consider these suggestions:

Use clear water to rinse your breasts when bathing so that the protective oils produced by the new oil glands are not washed away.

If you want to toughen your nipples to make the nursing transition easier and less painful, you can use a soft washcloth to rub them so that they get tougher. As you adjust to this texture, you can graduate to something rougher so that your nipples are not quite as sensitive by the time you start to nurse your baby.

If your breasts are swollen or uncomfortable, you can put a cool ice pack inside a wash cloth and hold it against the side of the breast to bring down the swelling or take a warm shower to soothe the tissue.

During your second trimester, your doctor may recommend other tests to monitor the growth of your baby.

Amniocentesis is usually performed between 13 and 18 weeks, sometimes later in the pregnancy depending on the situation. The doctor will numb your abdomen and insert a long needle into the amniotic sac. There is no risk to your baby.

The fluid drawn from the sac can tell the doctor about abnormalities or problems. If you are over 35, your doctor may recommend this test to be sure that your pregnancy is progressing normally.

A percutaneous umbilical blood sampling (PUBS or cordiocentesis) helps your doctor tell if your baby suffers from specific diseases like sickle cell disease and hemophilia. In this test, a needle is also passed through your abdomen, into your uterus.

But in this case, the doctor will draw a small sample of blood from the umbilical cord.

Sometime around week 15 of your pregnancy your doctor may suggest an ultrasound or sonogram, to look at the size of your baby and determine whether your pregnancy is on schedule.

An ultrasound is painless, but you do have drink and hold a lot of water, so you may be a bit uncomfortable. The technician will use a handheld device and slide it back and forth across your abdomen, to produce an image of your baby from high frequency sound waves.

If you are still exercising by the end of your 2nd trimester – good for you!

Just remember not to push yourself until you are out of breath or exhausted. Take breaks and allow yourself the luxury of adjusting to your new size and shape.

Avoid exercise that strains your lower back or legs, or exercises that require you to lie flat on the floor.

Instead of riding a bike in the street, consider riding a stationary bike so that your balance and shifting center of gravity do not cause you to fall.

You can exercise by scrubbing the floor or taking a power walk to the post office or corner market.

This is also a good time to start your Kegel exercises, named after Dr. Arnold Kegel. Kegel exercises strengthen your pelvic floor and prepare you for delivery, and you can do them anywhere.

Tighten and release the muscles on your pelvic floor as if you were trying to stop the flow of urine.

The name of the muscle you are tightening and releasing is 'pubococcygeus' (PC) and it goes from your pubic bone to your tailbone. Pregnancy can weaken this muscle and cause you to leak urine when you laugh, cough or strain.

One study reported that 50% of pregnant women had symptoms of 'bladder weaknesses during and after pregnancy.

But the Kegel exercise doesn't just keep you dry, it keeps your baby's head in the best position for labor and delivery, so it is doubly important.

Don't make the mistake of tightening your entire lower abdomen, thighs and/or buttocks. Be sure you isolate and specify the muscle by thinking of tightening the muscle you would tighten to stop urinating.

Kegel is easy to do, and you can do it whenever you THINK about doing it; at the grocery store or at work. Start with 10 to 25 cycles, a few times a day, and work your way up to 100 squeezes a day.

Sometime during this trimester, you will probably notice a change in your hair and skin texture. Some women report oilier or drier than normal hair and skin, and some even say their hair gets straighter or curlier.

Some women also report that their hair grows faster, and that their skin is more sensitive when they are pregnant.

The glands that produce oil in your body will increase or decrease production depending on your hormonal balance.

For some women, the second trimester of their pregnancy signals the best 'hair days' of their lives.

While there is no evidence that coloring your hair can hurt your baby, if you want to stay away from harsh dyes or permanent solutions you can ask your stylist to use techniques that do not directly impact the scalp and provide only highlights or temporary color.

But remember that your new hair texture may 'take' dye in a different way than your old hair once did. So, be ready for anything!

This is the time most women buy a new pair of larger shoes. Yes, your feet do grow during pregnancy and may grow as much as one full size. Choose comfortable, slip on, supportive shoes and wear maternity pantyhose if you find your legs getting tired or swollen during the day.

Sometime between week 18 and week 22 of your pregnancy you will feel your baby moving in the womb. If you are overweight it may take longer for you to feel movement. And sometimes the placenta is located toward the front of the uterus so it is harder to feel the baby move until it gets larger.

In time your baby will kick and move and the feeling will be so sharp that it is hard to ignore. By the 23rd week, your baby is much more sensitive to sound and touch coming from the outside so you can expect that you will get a response if something startling happens.

A baby's activity will increase up to 10 times the normal level when mom is under emotional stress. So if you have a near miss car accident or something startles you, you will notice your baby's reaction, a well.

Pregnancy hormones will also act on your emotions so be prepared to feel overly emotional about everyday things and to have some strange and emotional dreams when you sleep. This is all normal. However, IF you experience any signs of depression or mental disturbance, be sure to talk to your doctor immediately.

In general, the second trimester will be easier than the first and the third. By now you are used to coping with heartburn, back pain, headaches, fatigue and other symptoms and you have adjusted your lifestyle to accommodate your pregnancy.

Be sure to drink plenty of water, eat right, keep your blood sugar in check and get plenty of rest. If you work or go to school, be sure to get your feet up as often as possible to keep your back and legs from bothering you.

The Third Trimester

As you pass through your third trimester, your body is changing more quickly.

Nearly all pregnant women get stretch marks, those streaks that appear on your stomach and thighs as your body expends.

There is no 'cure' for stretch marks, but they do fade after pregnancy.

Keep your skin hydrated by drinking plenty of water and use a good non-greasy moisturizer on your abdomen, and legs to prevent dryness and keep the worst of the stretch marks at bay. This moisturizing will also decrease itching which many pregnant women report during late pregnancy.

You may also see varicose or spider veins during your late pregnancy. These most commonly appear around your ankles and feet where you have lots of swelling, but they can appear in other places as well.

Wear maternity pantyhose and put your feet up often to reduce swelling.

If you find that you perspire more easily, use powder and wear well-ventilated clothing so that you don't get a rash or increase perspiration and odor during these late months.

About one in 150 women encounter pruritic urticarial papules (PUPP) during late pregnancy. These are red, itchy patches that usually appear on your stomach. Talk to your doctor to get a good cream to treat these patches.

Be careful not to get overheated or hold your breath for long periods of time when you are in late pregnancy. This will affect the blood vessels in your body which are already working overtime to provide oxygenated blood to you and to your baby.

Every woman complains about sagging breasts in late pregnancy and after pregnancy but you should know that gravity will take its toll even if you never had a child.

So relax!

There is no way, short of surgery, to make your breasts small and perky again but you should acknowledge the changes by wearing a supportive bra, and you can help yourself by using good poster and by lifting arm weights and doing arm exercises to give your chest muscles more tone.

You will want to wait until after you deliver to do this, though!

As your baby grows to about 28 weeks in the womb, she/he will run out of room to play and kick and you may notice a bit less activity. Someplace around week 35 or 36, your baby will turn into the 'heads down' position for birth and you may notice that the bulge in your abdomen 'drops' lower.

This will put even more pressure on your bladder and you will feel like you are running to the bathroom every five minutes, though you will welcome the relief of pressure on your rib cage.

Though your baby's movement has slowed, you should still feel the baby moving about 10 times within a 2 hr. period. If you do not feel movement during a reasonably long time period and you are concerned, call your doctor immediately.

But be aware that there may be no problem. Your baby may be sleeping during that time. If your doctor feels the need to monitor your child, he may suggest a non-stress test to determine the baby's heart rate and ensure that the baby is not in any distress.

During your late pregnancy, your doctor may advise a urine test or a glucose tolerance test if you have a family history of diabetes or if your blood sugar has been high.

In these last few months you may notice more problems with digestion and heartburn, simply because there is less space for your body to do its work.

Be sure to drink plenty of water and try to eat small amounts more often so you are not overstuffed. Take a walk after you eat to stimulate digestion.

Some pregnant women sleep in a 'propped' position or support themselves with pillows to allow better digestion and to relieve discomfort.

During your last weeks of pregnancy you will probably align your sleep patterns to those of your baby. By now, you are hopefully on maternity leave and if you have difficulty getting enough rest, you may want to try to nap when you feel the need.

Your baby is likely to squirm when you lie down. This is because he can adjust and take a bit more space for himself when you are lying down, so let him get comfortable after you get comfortable.

In order to improve your sleep, eat a light meal at dinner time so you don't feel stuffed, and try taking a walk after dinner.

Take a warm (not extremely hot) bath before bed and stretch a little to loosen your muscles. Listen to relaxing music and be sure the room is dark so you can sleep.

It is common for pregnant women to experience painless Braxton-Hicks contractions during the last few months of pregnancy. These do not signal labor, but instead will fade and disappear.

Some changes you WILL note that indicate you are getting closer:

Your doctor may report that your cervix is thinner and is starting to dilate. This doesn't mean you are going to the hospital at that moment, though. You may wait for a few days before it is time.

You may see a small amount of pink or red jelly-like stain indicated that the plug that seals off the mouth of the uterus has come loose. Labor may still be a few days off but let your doctor know that this has happened.

Remember that your baby will give your body the signal when he/she is ready to be born. A complex set of hormonal changes will take place to soften the cervix and start contractions that will push the baby out into the world.

If you go well beyond your due date, your doctor may suggest keeping a 'kick count' to see how active your baby is over a certain number of hours. Or he may suggest a sonogram to measure amniotic fluid, and fetal activity.

If you are past 40 weeks gestation, your doctor MAY suggest that you induce labor, though most doctors prefer to wait for the baby's signal. However, if your baby is in distress or if your pregnancy is protracted and causing your health problems, induction may be necessary.

Your doctor will check you into the hospital and give you medication to start or enhance contractions and to get the process moving.

CHAPTER 9 - PREPARING FOR THE DAY

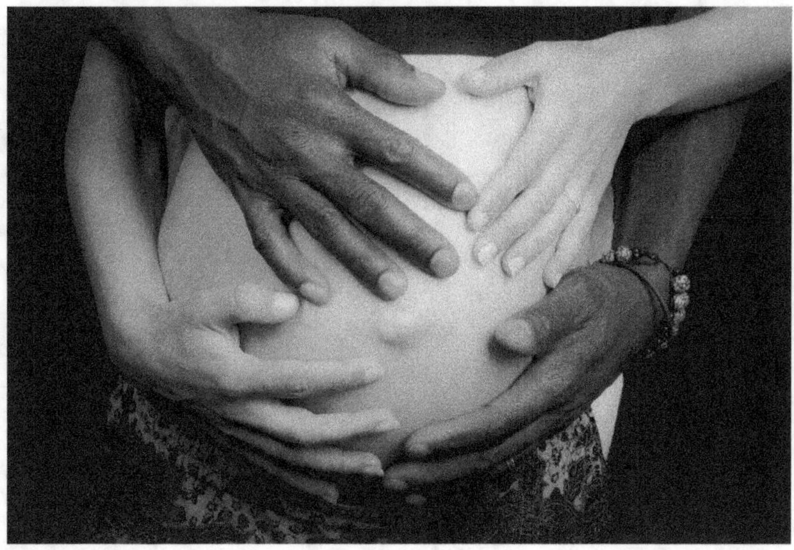

During your second or third trimester, you should begin to look at the hospitals or birthing centers with whom your health care professional is associated.

If you have a choice of facilities, take a tour of the maternity area to decide which facility you prefer. You can arrange a tour by calling the hospital or birthing center.

We'll give you some suggestions on questions to ask and things to look for that will make your delivery day easier and ensure that there are no surprises.

Patient's Rights and Informed Consent

Remember that you have rights as a patient and get a copy of the hospital or birthing center privacy and patient rights brochures. Read it thoroughly and be sure to ask your doctor and the staff at the facility any questions you may have about these standards.

Any medical procedures, tests, medications or other action that is administered to you during your delivery and your time in the hospital requires 'informed consent'.

In other words, the staff must explain what they are doing and WHY they are doing it and you have the right to refuse treatment if you wish.

You doctor, midwife and medical staff MUST tell you about the benefits AND the risks of any procedure or action they plan to take.

The consent form you sign when you are admitted does not mean you can't change your mind about a specific procedure or issue, so ask questions and know your rights.

Understand that your doctor is bound by oath and by law to care for you and your baby so if you refuse a procedure that she feels is necessary she may choose to proceed with this procedure anyway and she is legally protected if she does so. You will have to sort out the legality and the outcome after delivery!

You also have a right to ask for a second opinion about your treatment but in an emergency, there may not be time to call for another doctor and get that second opinion.

It is important to note that, in most cases, your pregnancy and delivery will proceed in a healthy manner and you will never be faced with these kinds of life and death decisions.

But, even for the small decisions where you have options, you do have the right to get a second opinion or to refuse what your doctor recommends, so it is important that you know your rights. Your doctor, midwife and medical staff are there to help you, not to hurt you, and in most cases, you won't face any significant disagreement.

Once you have chosen your birthing facility, get familiar with the procedures and the layout of the facility so that you can relax and be calm on the day of your delivery.

Remember, if you know where you are going and what is going to happen to you, you are less likely to be stressed over the small details.

And you will need your energy and focus to attend to your labor and delivery.

Things to Know about the Maternity Care Facility

If you are going to write a 'birth plan' that indicates your wishes for how you want your labor and delivery managed, ask to have this plan put on file and find out whether you need to bring another copy when you come to the hospital (just in case they can't find the one you gave them).

We'll give you some details about drafting a birth plan in a minute.

Also, find out if they will FOLLOW this plan, presuming there are no emergencies or special circumstances. Does your chosen hospital have policies they must follow for all patients in labor? If so, you should find out what they are so that you can take them into consideration when you write your birth plan.

Find out about nursing care as well. How many nurses are on duty in the birthing center or maternity area? How long are their shifts? How many patients does each nurse manage?

Ask about birth-related statistics: How many babies are delivered at this facility per year? How many are vaginal births (with or without medication), how many are C-sections?

How many births do they induce every year (be sure you talk to your doctor about his/her policies in this regard as well, so that you know you will be allowed ample opportunity to delivery before he recommends an induction).

Ask whether your hospital or facility is a teaching hospital where you may have students or residents treating you. If so, and if you are not comfortable with this, find out if you can refuse treatment by students and residents and how to do that, if necessary.

And ask how you will have to request a second opinion if you need one.

What devices does your hospital use to monitor your labor and your baby's progress during labor? Does this facility use continuous electronic fetal monitoring? If don't want this monitoring on a continuous basis, do you have the option of periodic monitoring?

If you are uncomfortable during labor and wish to refuse a pelvic exam, can you do so?

Does the birthing center or maternity wing have an obstetrical anesthesiologist on call in case you need one? Can you make an appointment to talk to an anesthesiologist before you go into labor so that you understand your options for pain medication and what will happen if you need a C-section?

Be sure you ask the anesthesiologist to explain the use of an epidural. What is it, how is it administered and how will it affect you during and after delivery? When is the epidural administered during labor? Is it always effective?

Talk to the staff and the anesthesiologist about the procedures for C-sections. How and when will the decision be made? Will your labor coach or partner be allowed to stay in the operating room with you?

Where is the procedure performed? Can you see the room in advance so you know what to expect? Where will you be moved after surgery and how long will stay in the recovery area? What kind of medication will they give you for pain?

Will you have IVs or a catheter and if so, when will they be removed? How will this procedure affect your ability to nurse and take care of your baby?

Prepare for Your Time after the Baby is Born

Take a tour of the nursery and find out if your baby will be allowed to stay in your room most of the day or if she/he will be brought to you at certain hours for feeding. What if you are not feeling well? Will the baby stay in the nursery temporarily or will the baby stay in your room?

Ask about special care facilities for your newborn. What if your baby is born prematurely or has a medical problem? Where is this special nursery? Can you take a tour of the facility and see what the equipment and nursing staff is like?

Neonatal Intensive Care Units (NICU) are very important if you have a child with special needs, so be sure you understand your options in this regard.

What is the visiting policy? Can you visit your baby at any time? Will you need to wear special gowns or clothing to go into the room?

Get a list of the routine vaccinations and procedures they plan for your baby: injections, tests, medications, etc.

And ask what each of these means so that you know what they are doing when the staff tells you they are about to perform a test or give your baby a shot.

If you have a boy, ask about the hospital policy regarding circumcision. Is this optional or do they automatically circumcise your child. Will your child receive pain medication for the circumcision and afterwards if necessary? If you are Jewish and you plan to have this done by a moile, be sure to let the hospital know this!

Lastly, find out how long your hospital stay will be for a normal vaginal delivery and for a C-section birth if required.

Now, take all these details and consider them for your birth plan. Make it specific so that your doctors and other medical staff don't have to guess if you are unable to discuss it with them.

The reason we suggest a birth plan is because it helps you to organize and consider your preferences and to ask all the right questions of your doctor and your hospital or birthing center staff so you are well prepared for your delivery.

Birth plans are not legal documents, but you should show yours to your doctor and get him to sign off on your plans to be sure you are being reasonable in your expectations.

Include information in your birth plan about whether you want induction, amniocentesis, IVs, heparin locks, enemas, epidurals, medications or narcotics, whether you want to eat or drink, use a birthing tub, move around or walk during labor, how you wish to be monitored (continuous or periodic), whether you want your doctor to use forceps, whether you want 'self-directed' pushing vs. doctor directed pushing.

Keep your birth plan short and easy to read (try to type it if you can so no one has to struggle over poor hand writing). Hospital staff will not read the document if it is too long and wordy. Describe what you want and what you don't want!

Your birth plan can also include what happens after delivery: Do you want your husband to cut the umbilical cord, and hold the baby first? Will your baby receive medication or vaccine, will she be breast fed or bottle fed? What happens if your baby needs special care?

When you think about what you want and what you don't want you are more likely to talk to your doctor about all the crucial requirements before you get to the hospital. And there is often no time to have this discussion during labor.

Birth plans can have disadvantages. Some doctors and medical staff do not appreciate being told what you want, but in that case, you may be using the wrong staff.

If you have a 'testy' health care professional on your hands – but one you would like to keep because of their knowledge and skills – be prudent about how you approach your birth plan.

Talk to them first about the fact that you are thinking of doing one and ask for their input. That will get them engaged. After you've done the birth plan ask them to look at it and give you feedback.

Be willing to be flexible and reasonable. Don't feel you have to control every detail. Most doctors and hospital staff are reasonable enough to work with you if you approach them in a polite and respectful manner.

Now that you have drafted your birth plan, there are a few other things you'll want to ask your hospital or birthing center staff to be prepared for going home with your baby.

Ask if your birthing center or hospital offers 'after care' visits from nurses, lactation consultants or other health care professionals after you have been discharged from the facility.

And be sure you find out about classes or support groups for new parents. Most facilities offer these on site and others will recommend a community-based program that will help you learn basic skills like bathing your infant.

Some groups, like the La Leche League, provide support for nursing mothers.

And there are even support group round tables where new parents can share their excitement and concerns with other new parents and get answers from a skilled, knowledgeable facilitator.

Chapter 10 - What to Do When in Labor Pain

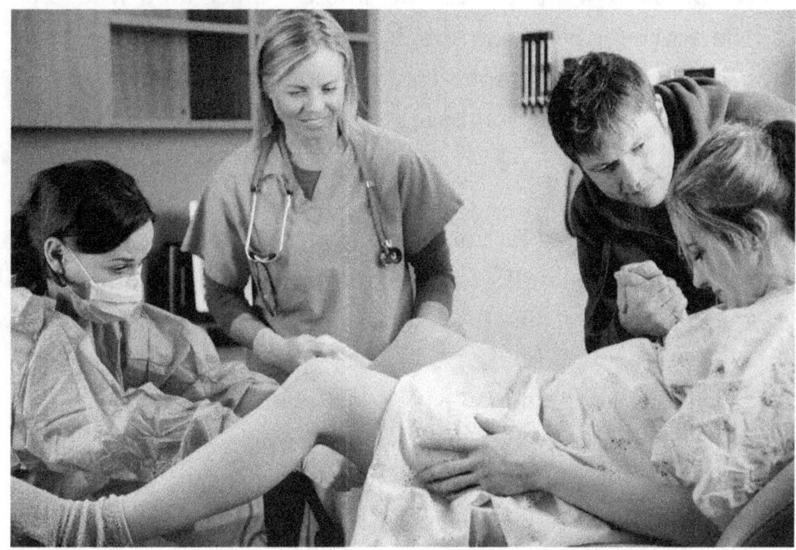

The waiting is over. You have finally reached the big day!

You should know that only about one in ten pregnant women experience the legendary 'breaking of the waters' as a first sign of impending birth.

If you are one of those women, you may feel a slow trickle that is only enough to dampen your underwear or you may wake up to a wet sheet in the morning. Rarely is there a dramatic gush of water.

The water from your amniotic sac has a slightly salty smell and it is clear and a bit sticky with some flecks. If your amniotic fluid is cloudy or green, tell your doctor this.

Labor contractions do not start right away, but they will usually appear somewhere between 24 and 48 hours after your amniotic fluid is released.

In any case, you should call your doctor to let him know that your 'water has broken'.

He will probably want you to come into the office for a visit so he can determine where you are in your labor schedule. He will probably apply an antiseptic cream around the opening to your uterus to be sure that you have protection against infection until your baby is born.

While you are waiting for your contractions to start, take showers, not baths, and don't allow anything into your vagina other than your doctor's sterile glove!

Before you go into you may have some diarrhea or vomiting. This doesn't always happen but it will happen in many women. If you do experience these symptoms, your labor will typically begin within 12-24 hrs. after the onset of nausea or diarrhea.

DO NOT try any herbal remedies or other things to induce labor on your own!

The following symptoms do not signal labor but may indicate a medical problem. You should call your doctor immediately if you experience any of these:

• Abdominal pain as opposed to uterine pain

• Vaginal bleeding

•Absence of fetal movement for 24 hours (after the fifth month of your pregnancy)

• Dim or blurry vision, or severe or constant headache

• Severe swelling of eyelids, hands or face during last trimester

• Persistent, severe vomiting

When your labor starts, you will know that you are not having the old standby Braxton Hicks contractions you have had during your pregnancy.

Remember that these contractions are relatively painless and last only 30-60 seconds. True labor contractions are longer and more regular and will not go away.

They will increase in strength and severity as your labor progresses and they will get closer together as your delivery draws near.

You don't have to run to the hospital or birthing center at the first sign of labor. You are more likely to remain calm and comfortable at home and you will usually have plenty of time to get there.

If your partner or labor coach is at a distance from you or the hospital, let them know you have started labor and get someone to sit with you for a while if it will make you make comfortable.

Allow plenty of time to get to the hospital if you live in a city or if you are leaving around rush hour.

If this is your first baby you may find that you are more uncomfortable during the first part of labor than during the last part. For experienced mothers, the end of the labor cycle seems to be more difficult. Whatever the case, don't panic. If you have taken a course for natural childbirth, you don't have to start your breathing and child birth strategies right away.

Just relax and wait until you need them!

You may have another 10 or 12 hours before you deliver and you want to your strength for the final sprint. Rest and drink plenty of water. You can even eat a little if you find you have an appetite. Just don't overload your stomach.

Eat healthy food like protein and vegetables or whole grain bread or just nibble on crackers and fruit.

If you find you want to take a bath, be sure you have help to get you in and out of the tub at home!

You should contact your doctor to let them know that labor has started.

She will probably tell you to call back when your contracts are about one minute in length and about five minutes apart.

If you are still not sure whether your labor is 'real', give yourself this mental test:

False Labor (prodromal) or Braxton-Hicks Contractions

Remember that Braxton- Hicks contractions stay at about the same intensity over the time have them. They are the same an hour ago as they are now and they only last 30 seconds or so. These contractions will go away if you walk move or change positions. There is no significant discomfort or pain associated with these contractions. You may have a backache.

The less common 'prodromal labor, is a kind of 'dry run' or practice labor that can cause lower back pain with contractions.

These contractions may feel more real than Braxton-Hicks, but they will not get closer together or stronger over time. If you get up and move around they will sometimes disappear completely.

Labor Contractions

Get progressively stronger and last longer as the hours go by. They also get closer together as your labor progresses.

There is significant discomfort with these contractions, and nothing you do seem to change that. You can move, walk or change positions and the contractions are still strong and predictable and painful.

You have pain in the back and in your abdomen (like a 'too tight' seatbelt or band around your stomach that keeps getting tighter).

IMPORTANT: If at any time you feel a significant pressure to push, you should get to the hospital immediately, and forget the leisurely labor at home! If you can feel a bulge or firm protrusion between your legs at the mouth of your cervix, you should not try to make it to the hospital. Have someone call 911 and get yourself comfortable on your bed with extra clean towels or a clean (old) comforter underneath you. Or, if you are more comfortable on the floor, be sure you have plenty of clean padding underneath you and relax and breathe until the ambulance and EMTs arrive.

When you are ready to go to the hospital, don't try to go alone if you can help it. Have someone take you, call a cab or call an ambulance if you must.

When you get to the hospital on the day of delivery, be sure you ask if they have a copy of the birth plan. If not, have another copy ready to give them, and repeat your primary and most important requests then and there so that you remind the staff of what you want.

During labor your cervix will become thinner and more open. If you are a first time mother, this may take 10 hours or more. If you have already had a child it may take only 2-3 hours. Your doctor will refer to this dual process as 'effacing' and 'dilating', and he will use your progress to determine how soon you may give birth.

The thinning of the cervix (effacement) is noted as a percentage. If you are 25% effaced, you are only ¼ of the way there.

The widening of the opening in your cervix (dilation) is noted in centimeters or sometimes in 'fingers'. When your cervix is fully dilated it is about 10 centimeters across. Or your doctor may say you are '2 or 3 fingers' dilated, meaning your cervix is dilated by about 3-4 centimeters and still has a way to go.

As your labor progresses, contractions will get more intense and you will have shorter breaks between these contractions. But even at the longest point of your labor, these contractions never last more than 1.5 min. and you will typically have at least 30 sec between contractions.

Each contraction occurs in three stages:

• The Increment Phase (or start-up)

• The Acme Phase (the height of the contraction)

• The Decrement Phase (the contraction slows to a halt)

And you will get a brief rest in between each cycle.

Monica Libinski
The discomfort of labor is primarily from the pressure and weight of the baby's body putting pressure on your organs and body and traveling down through the birth canal, causing the hips to widen and the head and body to push against the cervix.

Stage 1 Labor

The upper half of your uterus becomes more dense and the lower half thinner so that it push against your baby to propel him/her down into the birth canal. Every time you have a contraction during this stage, your baby will move down and then come back up a little as it progresses through the narrow change in your pelvis.

Stage 2 Labor

This stage begins as soon as your cervix and uterus have completed their effacing and dilation processes. This stage is considerably shorter than the first stage and may last 20-60 minutes. Unless you are heavily medicated or you have had an epidural, she will feel like you MUST start pushing your baby out.

Try to resist this urge unless and until your doctor tells you to go ahead. And if you are going to push, try to control the 'when' on your own schedule, gently pushing with breathing in between so that you can go with what your body is telling you to do.

Because the uterus does most of the work, you may not have to push much at all and what doctors call the 'valsalv maneuver' or the 'purple push' will raise your blood pressure and tire you more quickly.

So, if your doctor asks you to push, ask him to do it on your own count as you are ready. Your baby will be born within the same time period and you and the baby will both be less stressed.

Once your baby is born your doctor will snip the umbilical cord (the umbilical cord is about 22 inches long, and looks rather like a spiral tube with a white membrane covering it), and your baby will become its own independent entity, no longer dependent on your body though certainly dependent on you as her new mother in this brave new world!

The doctor will then take the baby for a moment to clean out her mouth and record her vital statistics (weight, length, etc.). You will probably get a chance to hold the baby right after he has finished his work.

Remember that babies arrive on their own schedule, so your labor may be shorter or longer than someone else's. In most cases, this is just what is normal for you and for THIS baby – not necessarily what will happen in any subsequent births.

Before we finish talking about labor, we should note that you have one more thing to do before your delivery is over.

You have to expel the placenta (the amniotic sac that has nourished and cradled your baby while he/she has developed in your uterus).

During your pregnancy, the placenta is attached to the wall of your uterus with slender threads or roots and it gets its nourishment for your baby from your body.

It stores carbohydrates, minerals, protein, and fats and feeds them to your child through the umbilical cord, and it is the conduit for oxygen to your baby's body.

It also carries away waste matter and carbon monoxide which is then washed through your kidneys and out of your system.

At the time of your baby's birth, the placenta will be about 6-8 inches in diameter, about 1 inch thick and about one pound in weight.

After your baby is born, the placenta will detach itself from the uterine wall so you can 'deliver' it through the same channel from which your baby was born.

If you see the placenta while your doctor is delivering it, you will notice its rich red, kidney bean color and a texture that is squishy and sponge-like.

Your doctor will put the placenta in a bowl and examine it to be sure that it is intact and there are no fragments missing that may still be attached to the uterine wall.

Within hours after delivery, your uterus will shrink; reverting to almost normal size within ten days after your baby is born.

For about six weeks after delivery, you will experience some bleeding as your uterus cleans out the remaining fluid and other artifacts of your pregnancy. If this discharge has a foul or strange odor, call your doctor and let her know.

A few months after 'housekeeping' activities are completed, your ovaries will release another egg, and you are once again ready to 'make a baby'.

About the Author

Monica Libinski is a La Leche counsellor. She has helped thousands of women conceive naturally and keep their pregnancies healthy.

A midwife by profession, Monica has made it her personal responsibility to society to keep mothers and babies healthy. She is a mother herself and she understands the joys and pains of motherhood through first-hand experience.

www.ingramcontent.com/pod-product-compliance
Lightning Source LLC
Chambersburg PA
CBHW071019260726
48662CB00022B/598